Reiki Heal

The Book of Light

By Mark F Kalita

Reiki Heal

*A healing technique based on
the principle that anyone can
channel Reiki into their body
and activate natural healing
processes to restore physical
and emotional well-being.*

Table of Contents

FOREWORD

'Neither shall they say, 'Lo, it is here!' or 'Lo, it is there!' For behold, the Kingdom of God is within you.'
                                                  Luke 17:21

As long as I can remember, I have struggled with the conflicted nature of religions and what I knew to be true within me. It wasn't until I began to use Reiki that things became clear to me. When I allowed Reiki into my life, or so I thought, things began to change for me.

Little did I know that Reiki has been with me - my whole life. In 2001, I didn't discover Reiki, I rediscovered something that I held throughout my entire life, but didn't know about.

You see, this Universal Life Energy (ULE) that is at the center of the practice of Reiki, is always with us. It is a part of life itself.

It has been called many things throughout the ages and within the ancient religions, but those are just words. Words cannot describe the indescribable.

The above quote from the Christian Bible, shows just one of the many ways this ULE has been described throughout the ages. Yet, in almost all of these religions, this ULE is referred to as the 'Light'.

In the Pure Land sect of Buddhism, they await Amida Buddha, the Buddha of Infinite Light and Life.

In the Qu'ran, it is written that the UMMI will appear upon the Earth. He will be known by the Light that he carries. It is told that he who follows the UMMI will have success.

In Christianity, Jesus was of the Light. It is this Light that surrounds many of the Spiritual manifestations expressed in those texts. From his baptism with John to his followers finding the Light after his death. This Light is central to the Christian doctrine.

From the earliest stories in the Tanakh, Judaism has a strong tradition of this Light from God. From the first emanation of Light in Genesis to the Prophets talking about a coming Light, the Light of God is preeminent.

Isaac Luria, a sixteenth century Rabbi and founder of Lurian Kabalah, wrote a number of poems that describe his views of God and existence. I have included his poem "Tree of Life" in Appendix A.

These stories continue across the face of the Earth. Every ancient tradition has the stories of this universal Light that permeates all things. Not just from one tradition, but from within all major religious and indigenous traditions.

The Native American Tribes have many stories of the ULE and the Great Spirit. The ONEness that their tribes held modern society has yet to find.

Yet, when I talk about Reiki, people get all flustered. Because Reiki uses Sanskrit and Japanese symbols, there are religions that have warned their adherents against Reiki.

Reiki is not a religion, religiously based or affiliated with any religious tradition.

Yet, Reiki is affiliated with all religious traditions as it is the Light of the ULE that Reiki helps facilitate the flow of.

It is called the 'hidden manna' in the "Book of Revelations" for a very good reason. This Light, the ULE, heals.

It is not the Reiki or the Reiki practitioner that heals, it is the Light of God that heals.

When I say that "I Reiki Heal", I mean that I facilitate the Reiki by being a channel to the Light and by removing blocks within my clients. These blocks could be physical, emotional, mental or Karmic in nature. When the blocks are removed, the Light is able to flow freely.

When the Light is blocked sickness occurs. Either physical manifestations, through emotional episodes or other symptoms of unbalance.

Life can even be shortened by a life of major blockages.

When the Light becomes unblocked, balance and healing can take place. The body becomes healthier. And, if these blocks are removed early enough, life can be extended.

How does Reiki do it differently from other spiritual techniques that try to help facilitate the flow of Light?

Through plain language, a tradition of healing and a process to remove the blocks so that the Light can flow smoothly.

I believe that many of the world religions had a system of healing like Reiki. Because of the changing beliefs and attitudes, these 'secret' teachings were lost. Unfortunately, when they were lost, the adherents to these various religious traditions didn't even know anything was lost.

Then, in the early part of the last century, a system to unblock the Light was rediscovered. From within meditation, inspiration was given to a man to resurrect an ancient tradition.

This system became known as Usui Reiki. Sensei Usui was Japanese, so 'Reiki' is the word he knew for the Light that he saw.

Reiki simply means "Universal Life Energy" in Japanese. It is this ULE that I facilitate. I use the traditions found within Usui Reiki to do that.

And, so can you!

This ULE is at the center of you. This ULE is at the center of all of us. In this book, "I Reiki Heal: The Handbook of Light", I will attempt to show you, through my experience, that these techniques are universal.

Anyone can practice Reiki, as everyone has the Light within them. You are utilizing the ULE right now. It flows through you just as sure as your blood flows.

Yet, unblocking the ULE within your body is a multifaceted gemstone. There are so many facets of you that could potentiality block the ULE. From current relationships to relationships in past lives, the greater work has to be done by you to understand your lessons.

A Reiki practitioner only shines the Light so that you might see.

And, that is why I am writing this book – to shine the Light on a knowledge and a compassion that has gifted me with being an open circuit for the Light. It is this 'proper knowledge' and 'proper compassion' that is at the center of many religious traditions who speak of finding this Light.

In the Pure Land sect of Buddhism, this shows as the Bodhisattvas of Knowledge and Compassion. Upon attainment, one receives the 'Infinite Light' of Amida.

In Judaism, this shows as the Two Anointed Ones - the King and the Priest.

I will simply call it what it is:

'The understanding of the Infinite ONE, the Intelligent Infinity and the Light and Love that flows through all of existence.'

The contents of this book, "I Reiki Heal: The Handbook of Light" is not taught in any Reiki Tradition. This book is the 'Knowledge' and 'Compassion' that I use to connect with the Light. I have found that this 'Knowledge' has strengthened me in Reiki and has opened up new gifts within the three natures of the ONE – omnipresent, omnipotent and omniscient.

As this 'Knowledge' and 'Compassion' has helped me heal, I hope that you allow "I Reiki Heal: Handbook of Light" to be the beginning of your road in finding peace and Light in the ONE.

Chapter 1
Light

All that is known, and unknown, throughout the entire expanse of space is a singular entity functioning as a super-intelligence with dominion over all things. The children of the Earth have had many names for this Creator throughout history. Many of these names have run counter to the unity of life. These names have been used to exert power and dominion over others. In the simplest terms, let this Creator be known as the 'ONE'.

I use the word ONE, for that is the label of an understanding within our language and vernacular. Other words may be used to describe the Creator, yet none can even begin to fully explain the unexplainable. These are just words found within languages, not a name. The true understanding of the ONE is difficult to define as the ONE is incomprehensible and no word has come close to the true understanding of the Creator.

ONE seems to fit better than any other word to describe the super-intelligence at the core of ALL.

It is in this ONE that all things are.

We are ONE people.

Existence, and all that is within it, can be unified into this ONE.

The ONE is, was, and will ever be.

The ONE is all around us, within us and drives us on our journey through life. The ONE is all that is seen and unseen. The Infinite energies of the ONE hold Creation together in Love and Light. The three natures of the ONE are; omnipotent, omnipresent, and omniscient.

Omnipotent has the meaning of 'All Powerful'. This can be relayed as the ability to change this material manifestation. This appears as healing primarily, but can also be related to other changes in the physical plane.

Omnipresent has the meaning of 'Ever Present'. This can be relayed as the ability to be everywhere at any time.

Omniscient has the meaning of 'All Knowing'. This can be relayed as intuition, foreknowledge, prophecy and all-seeing.

The guiding tenet within this realm is:

All is of the ONE, is the ONE, and is the ONE's.

All of the Earth, and all therein, is of the ONE.

This understanding gives greater meaning to the previous communications of the Love, Light and knowledge of the ONE.

Love the ONE with all your heart, and with all your soul, and with all your mind.

Love your neighbor as yourself.

To this I add - Love the Earth and all of existence as if it were your own.

For, if everything is of the ONE, is the ONE, and is the ONE's, give all of existence your unconditional love. Care for that which has been entrusted to you. Be as gentle stewards to all of Creation so that these gifts of the ONE may be safeguarded for all generations of our ONE family upon the Earth.

These are the primary laws by which our existence is bound. And, since this understanding of the ONE is a truth, it does not require you to convert, or accept, any religious tradition. When you have understanding of this truth, you learn to naturally, and completely, submit to the ONE, while you gradually awaken to the truth that you are being held in a closed system of Love and Light - the unity of ONE.

We are all of the ONE, within the ONE, and are subtlety separated from the ONE by the love of the ONE.

The highest aspect of this understanding is unconditional love for the ONE, and all of existence.

When a person can achieve this state of unconditional love for everything that exists through the understanding of the ONE, that person becomes enlightened in the knowledge of the ONE.

The goal of all beings is to live in the unity of ONE and emulate the Love and Light of the ONE.

It is through this goal that the ONE gave us the gift of separation, so that we would know the ONE, fashion ourselves after the ONE, and return to the ONE.

This is the knowledge of the gift of separation and of the ONE.

With the gift of separation into self and other-self, individual beings have the ability to see outside of self and know Love of other-self, Love of existence and Love of the ONE.

It is with this Love for all things that we find our way back to the unity of the ONE.

Our journey begins with separation from the ONE. We then learn the lessons of this separation. Eventually we find our way back to the ONE and are united with the ONE in the pure Love and Light of the ONE.

And, as our earthly family comes together as ONE, we will find everlasting peace. We will learn to live in unity. We will learn to live as the ONE intended.

ONE, as simplistic as it may seem, is a unifying word that tells so much more about the true nature of the universe than all of the divisive words that have been used to describe the Creator in the past.

This ONE, in it's current waking state, is on a discovery of self. As the ONE awoke, a self realization occurred that the ONE could not know of self completely without the interaction of other-self. This journey of discovery stimulated Creation. Through this creation of the vast material universe, the many scenarios of self and other-self began.

The eternal moment gave way so that this experience could manifest. The ONE, within the Infinite, wished to explore the Finite, as well as Free Will. Throughout many realms, individual entities are spun off of this original soul to experience the complexities of self and other-self.

All experience, the total sum of consciousness from each soul-being within all realms, becomes a memory of the ONE. As recorded within the ONE, ultimately, these records are also available to individual entities while their current incarnation is tuned to the tenets of ONE.

As every other-self is spun off of the ONE, so too does that other-self begin a journey to assist the ONE in discovery of self. The purpose of an individual soul-being is to find their way back to the unity of this original soul, the ONE.

Our goal is to find our way back to the ONE.

Understanding that everything is of the ONE, we realize that unconditional Love for All is at the core of the ONE. Our choices within each incarnation are paramount in finding our way back to the ONE. This is the true nature of our spiritual lives.

The 'Divinity' of the ONE extends naturally to all other-selves as being 'Divine', as well as to all of Creation.

The Earth, and all that is upon it, is supported in but a fraction of the ONE. The ONE is within us. The ONE is all around us. The plants, animals, fish, mountains, rivers, oceans and plains are all part of the ONE.

All living entities within this realm carry the energies of life within. These energies emanate from the ONE, are part of the ONE and can be utilized by a soul-being for the betterment of the ONE. Within the center of all living entities does this ONE reside, orchestrating their movements and offering guidance back to the unity of the ONE. This is the Light and Love of the ONE.

This material manifestation is comprised of forces seen and unseen. As there is a 'spiritual' world just as real as the 'material' world. These constructs were first revealed in ancient texts that described these 'spiritual' energies as 'Light' and the causal reaction when these 'Light' energies are used. This Light of the ONE can be measured and shown to be as real as the 'material' energies we are familiar with.

Yet, by being a manifestation of intelligent design, the seat of spirit, or soul, within all entities is the connection to the causal effects of this Light. Our bodies, or Temples, act as both antennae and source for the Light. Every Human being is designed in this image.

By these facts, very Human is 'Divine' and sacred to the ONE. The ONE resides within all, as all reside within the ONE. The Light and Love of the ONE flows naturally through all beings in this realm.

All were made as male and female, of tribes and kingdoms so that we may come together as ONE community. If you look to the east and the west, there you will see the ONE looking back at you, waiting for you to understand these basic tenets of unity.

Find the ONE and you will find peace, not only in your life, but also within the greater world. That is the true eventuality of our ONE family upon the Earth. Finding peace through the unity of the ONE is where we are all walking as a family – together.

We are ONE people on this ONE Earth under the ONE Creator.

As much as there are differences in all of us, we should all see that there are similarities that unite us all.

We all walk on the same Earth.

We all see from the light of the same Sun.

We all breath the same air.

We all look to the Earth for sustenance.

We all drink of the same waters.

We all bleed with the same blood.

We are all of the same family.

We are ONE.

As many times as it has been said in the past and as many times as we have shared these common truths, the story will never change – we are ONE.

All of our family must be taught this understanding of existence, as it is the core of all that is known. Find the Love for All so that together we can build unity to safeguard all generations of our ONE family.

This is the road map, but it is up to you, each and every person upon the Earth, to travel the road of Light towards peace, truth and altruistic lovingkindness on your own. It is a choice that you must make for yourselves – be as ONE in the Light and Love so that the blessings of the ONE will shower down upon you.

And, those new gifts that will be bestowed upon you will be the blessings of the ONE that were promised to your forebears. These blessings of health, well being, and life for evermore can only be earned through living within the righteousness of Love for All.

This is the knowledge of the Light and Love of ONE.

Chapter 2
Temple

Your physical body is your Temple which holds your mind and spirit. Temples are a sacred gift of the ONE and must be held in that sacredness. All of our family, as all have a Temple, should be held as sacred. The ONE gave you this life and the gift of your Temple to cherish and behold the existence of this realm and of the ONE. Within this incarnation, you have been given the gift of separation so that you would know the ONE.

Imagine now, if you could, without the gift of separation you would be part of the ONE and would not know the ONE except through the knowledge of self. Within the gift of separation, you are now able to have understanding of both self and of other-self.

Imagine looking at your brother, your sister, your son, your daughter, your mother, your father, your neighbor, your friend, or your enemy and seeing the ONE within their eyes. See this other-self within all people of the Earth. Just as you have been given the gift of separation, so too have they.

As you are aware of other-self, you now have awareness of each other-self as still part of the ONE.

We are all children of the ONE.

Now, understand yourself and all other-selves as angels of the ONE. All other-selves are precious, loved and unique to the ONE. As you are 'Divine, so too are all children of the Earth 'Divine'.

As our Temples enter into this incarnation, a veil of forgetting shields our mind from the knowledge of past lives and experience. Time and space are seemingly linear within the illusion the entity comprehends. This veil is used to facilitate Free Will and the choices of Light and Darkness. If the veil was not present, the experience would be without meaning as all would be known.

It is through the design of the Temple that the ONE has given us likeness to the ONE. All Temples are, by their very nature, Creators alongside the ONE. Through understanding with the mind, interaction with other Temples and the Faith of spirit, entities may find unity within the ONE, fashion themselves after the ONE and join hands again with the ONE.

As an individual entity becomes tuned to Creation, unity reveals a likeness to the ONE.

The three spiritual natures that our Temples manifest of the ONE can be termed as being - Omnipotent, Omniscient, and Omnipresent. These three natures, when manifest in the Temples, can be used to benefit Creation.

The seven energy centers of our Temple allow us to tap into the infinite energies of the ONE when we learn to balance body, mind and spirit to the truth of the ONE. These energy centers can be used to connect to the ONE.

Also known as the Endocrine system, these seven systems are either blocked, or opened, to the energies of the ONE. Using mind and spirit together, as well as the interaction of other-selves, these energy centers can become open to the Infinite energies.

For example, the life span of Temples are shortened through negative influences that diminish the ONE. If the ONE were to be positively influenced by the actions of Temples, the life span of Temples would increase.

If Temples would all come together in ONE community that lived within the concept of Love for All, theoretically, the ONE would be replenished and provide the Temples a life without sickness or death.

Individual Temples can still look forward to better health and a seemingly longer life by living within the unity of ONE, but the greatest change is from ALL.

Respect of your Temple is paramount to your success. It is within the understanding that you are a "Divine Being" that you will find respect for your Temple.

Respect of other-selves is just as important. It is within knowing that other-selves are a "Divine Being" that will assist in balancing these energy centers.

For within Creation, it is the interaction of other-selves that will guide you to advancement towards the ONE. Love for All and Service to Others with a wisdom that compassion leads all beings to the Light of the ONE is the nature of life. This awareness opens the Temple to the Infinite energies abounding within the ONE.

Our separation from the ONE is a physical manifestation filled with obstacles and challenges. The seven energy centers are a bio-chemical source that not only fuels the Temple, but also gives the Temple emotional responses to situational experiences. Learning to balance these emotional responses, those lessons of Love for All, is the movement of the soul-being through life towards the ONE.

As these energy centers can be both source and receiver for the Infinite energies of the ONE, they must be fueled with a diet of proper nutrients. Not only does the Temple need proper Amino Acids for these energy centers, it also requires proper minerals. Yet, the intake of these nutrients should, as always, be absorbed with the core understanding found within Love for All.

It is the complete respect for the ONE through the Temple in which an entity will gain maximum benefit from the nutrients ingested. As 'all is of the ONE, is the ONE's and is the ONE', respect of the Earth and the animals of the Earth, within the understanding of Love for All, will aid the entity in the balance of the energy centers.

As the Earth was gifted to all by the ONE as our home, it was designed to be a vast garden that would fulfill our need for these nutrients. If properly utilized, the trees and plants found upon the Earth have the inherent potential to feed all beings. From fruit bearing trees to vegetables and herbs, these gifts of the ONE were meant to feed all life upon the Earth.

These, when ingested in a compassionate manner, will help the energy centers provide balance for the Temple. It is within this righteousness that the mind and spirit are awakened to the Love for All at the core of the unity of ONE.

As the energy centers are fueled properly, the work on the energy centers through the mind and spirit will be most beneficial.

Temples were created to aid in the interaction of self and other-self while learning the lessons of Service to Others. The nutritional aspects are only a portion of this balance. Being healthy is also found in movement and exercise. Keeping your Temple fit will help balance these energy centers. Temples were not created to be stationary. Nor were Temples created to be overweight.

Also, the ancient rites of our forebears knew the value in having long hair. The fine strands of long hair act as antennae to these energies of the ONE. While devices of ego have attempted to instill vanity to cut hair, growing the hair long will aid the Temple in the flow of the Light.

Vanity and power struggles against other-selves work against the Love for All at the core nature of the ONE. All other-selves are also of the ONE.

Always keep in mind this respect for your own Temple, as well as the Temples of other-selves. Practice an all compassionate Love which demands no expectation of return from any other-self, or from the world around you.

Be at peace with your Temple. Be at peace with the Temples of other-selves. Do not be a possession, nor try to possess. Do not judge. Give freely your forgiveness. Remember, that as the ONE is Love for All, so too should all Temples residing within the ONE emulate this.

When a Temple is balanced in Love for All through the energy centers, the Light of the ONE is able to flow. That is the design of our Temple. That is the likeness to the ONE that all soul-beings share.

As the mind and spirit come into balance through the seven energy centers of the Temple, connection to the Light becomes possible. More than anything else, the understanding that 'All is of the ONE, is the ONE and is the ONE's' will assist in this balance.

First, a Temple must balance their connection to the Earth. This base energy center opens when the Temple accepts and understands the Light. Be as ONE with the Earth. Walking barefoot upon the land will assist the Temple in realizing this base energy.

As this first energy center is related to the Earth, in the Temple it is associated with basic potentiality. It is associated with the connection to the ONE and needs to only be realized to be opened

Second, a Temple must balance their connection to their self. This second energy center abounds with the emotions and acceptance of self. Be at peace with your Temple. Be at peace with your mind. Find joy and love with who you are. You are a special and precious. You are ONE with the ONE.

Third, a Temple must balance the energy center that is associated with their ego. To balance this energy center, a being must find peace in interactions of self and other-self as they relate to Love for All. Live in altruistic lovingkindness. See the ONE in all other-selves eyes. Just as you have been given the gift of Separation and your Temple, so too have all other-selves.

To balance this energy center realize that all Temples are sacred to the ONE. Do not hold yourself over any other-self by plays of power or ownership. Do not judge any other-self. Do not engage in vanity or holding yourself above any other-self. The ego is strong in the Temple. This energy center draws on the ego and will correspondingly fuel the ego.

When the ego is tempered by altruistic lovingkindness this energy center becomes balanced. When there is understanding that all other-selves are sacred within the ONE, this energy center becomes balanced in the Light.

The fourth energy center is associated with universal love and compassion. Many ancient systems of balancing these energy centers relate this fourth energy center to the heart. Understanding Love for All and that 'all is of the ONE, is the ONE's, and is the ONE' will assist in the opening of this energy center. When an entity makes the choice of Love for All, this energy center will find balance in the Light.

When this energy center is balanced, the Temple can open the gateway to the Infinite Light of the ONE.

A Temple, when balanced through these first four energy centers, is ready to depart on the journey of self discovery within the Infinite Intelligence of the ONE. These first four energy centers are the most difficult to balance to the unity of ONE. Through faith and compassion, a soul-being must first give in submission to the truths of the ONE and then use this faith through interactions with all other-selves to find balance.

The fifth energy center opens up the Temple to both the incoming and outgoing Light of the ONE. With further development of the mind and spirit accepting self and other-self, a Temple allows open communication. Not only is giving communication vital to this energy center, but it is also important to accept communication from other-selves.

The sixth energy center within the Temple is balanced with an increased understanding of self and self worth. As the lessons of the ONE are understood, a Temple who knows self to be as Creator, a "Divine Being" to the ONE, will balance this energy center. It is through this energy center that the super-intelligence of the ONE is accessed. The Temple begins to be as ONE with the Light as this energy center is balanced.

Through faith of the ONE, this energy center opens the Temple to a spiritual inner guidance with a clarity found in the balance of the previous energy centers. Knowing that self is part of the ONE as the ONE resides within self allows the Temple to understand fully that they are a Light being within the ONE.

The final energy center, that of the seventh, is the sum of the previous six energy centers. Opened or closed, balance or unbalanced, this energy center relies on the balance of the Temple in total and of faith in the ONE as Infinite Creator.

Being ONE with all of Creation is the gift of this energy center. Without want or need, the self learns that all is provided for by the Light and Love of the ONE. As the child in the womb, so too are we held by the ONE.

As Creator along side of the ONE, the Temple will now fully understand the affect of positive and negative contributions to the unity of the ONE.

While the Temple relies on the previous six energy centers to activate the seventh, when the seventh is opened the Temple finds unity with the ONE and the Light. Through the seventh energy center, the wisdom of Light and Love appear to the Temple.

When a Temple is balanced, and the Light flows freely throughout the Temple, the blessings of the ONE become readily available to the Temple. Each in their own experience of the ONE, a Temple may find the three natures of the ONE available; the Omnipresent, the Omnipotent, or the Omniscient. These three natures help the Temple to strengthen the ONE providing a benefit to all of Creation and all other-selves.

When balanced Temples gather together within the understanding of the ONE and Love for All, great works can be accomplished as the Light of the ONE is multiplied exponentially.

While this is a complex study of the energy centers found in the Temple, the real work is found in the simplicity of Love for All and the acceptance of the ONE. To love, forgive, accept, and open the entire Temple in mind and spirit through Love for All is the only requirement in balancing these energy centers. It is in the unity of the ONE that the manifestation of experience teaches the soul-being lessons of Love for All. It is in this gathering of Light and Love through unity that we are the ONE.

Separation gives the ONE knowledge of self by knowing the finite through free will. Interaction between self and other-self allows the ONE to know self. Interaction between self and other-self allows self to know the ONE. Knowing the ONE allows self to become the ONE.

The veil creates the physical manifestation in which Temples reside to find their way back to the ONE. The interaction between self and other-self is the manifestation of experience. The giving of Love for ALL without expectation of return moves the Temple closer to unity. Within unity the Temple accepts self as the ONE. With the faith of the ONE, the Temple again becomes the ONE.

In you, in all of your self doubt, unworthiness and pains of separation, does the ONE reside, seeking your return to the Infinite. You are Light.

You are LOVE.

You are the ONE.

All other-selves are as you. You are as all other-selves. All are in unity residing in the ONE. Whether this is your understanding, or not, it does not diminish the fact that there is only the ONE.

All are a sacred and share the Light and Love of the ONE.

Faith in the ONE is the cornerstone of unity and of peace. From interactions between self and other-self to the interaction of nations and kingdoms, peace can be found by using the knowledge of the ONE. Once peace is found globally, our ONE family will have unity.

A single, basic principle will allow every Temple success in our journey through life – Love for All within Service to Others through an understanding and faith in the ONE will bring us into the Light!

Chapter 3
Path

Within this incarnation, we have been given the gift of separation so that we would know the ONE.

All is of the ONE, is the ONE and is the ONE's.

The ONE is, was, and will ever be.

The ONE is omnipotent, omnipresent, and omniscient.

These are the primary laws by which our existence is bound. And, since this understanding of the ONE is a truth, it does not require you to convert, or accept, any religious tradition. When you have understanding of this truth, you learn to naturally, and completely, submit to the ONE, while you gradually awaken to the truth that you are being held in a closed system of Light and LOVE which is the unity of the ONE.

We are all of the ONE, within the ONE, and are subtlety separated from the ONE by the love of the ONE.

The highest aspect of this understanding is unconditional love for the ONE, and all of existence.

When a person can achieve this state of unconditional love for everything that exists through the understanding of the ONE, that person becomes enlightened.

The goal of all beings is to live in this unity of ONE.

It is through this goal that the ONE gave us the gift of separation, so that we would know the ONE, fashion ourselves after the ONE, and return to the ONE.

It is with this LOVE for ALL things that we find our way back to the unity of the ONE.

Our journey begins with separation from the ONE. We then learn the lessons of this separation. Eventually we find our way back to the ONE and are united with the ONE in the pure Light and LOVE of the ONE.

Path of Being

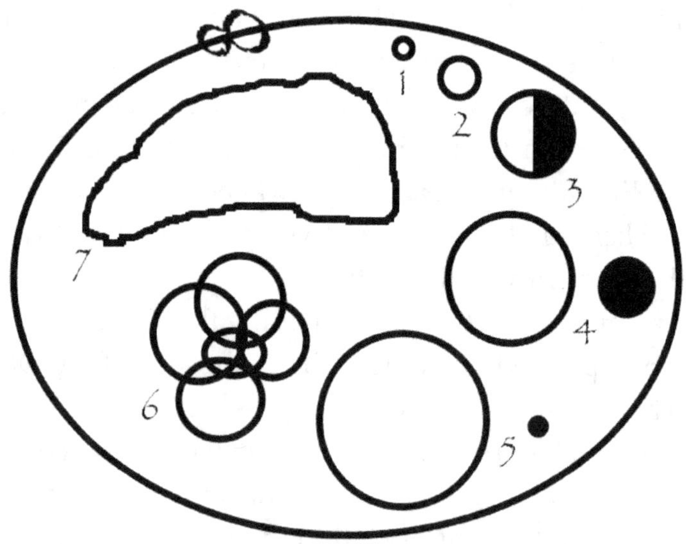

This is the 'Path of Being' that every soul-being takes through the ONE, or UNITY of existence.

This 'Path of Being' illustrates how ALL entities experience the Infinite ONE through this path of SEPARATION.

In this drawing, the OCTAVES of existence are numbered. This is our path through the realms of existence of ONE. They are shown as the 'Path of Being'.

The first Octave is the initial SEPARATION from the ONE, also known as the Original Soul. This is the beginning of the journey back to UNITY. While these young entities first deal with the SEPARATION, they are still united with the ONE in their material manifestation.

This is known to the children of the Earth as a plant. Like a tree that has it's roots within the Earth, an entity in this first OCTAVE is not yet fully separated from all that is. While still a living entity, this direct connection to the material manifestation of the ONE shelters the entity from the suffering inherent in their SEPARATION.

The second is the SEPARATION into BEING. As the individual entity is reborn into a seemingly separated life form, it has overcome the true SEPARATION from the Original Soul and is readied for a material manifestation in which it recognizes SELF. Still not fully aware of OTHER-SELF, this entity grows and learns individuality.

This is known to the children of the Earth as bird, animal, fish or other life form. The early lessons are that of BEING an individual entity. The later lessons are the nurturing of offspring, their first glimpses of other-self.

The Third OCTAVE is the knowledge of SELF and OTHER-SELF. This is known to us generally as SERVICE to SELF, or egotism, and SERVICE to OTHERS, or altruism. It is through this lesson in UNITY that we encounter POLARITY of BEING, that of GOOD or EVIL.

This is the realm of BEING that the children of the Earth currently reside.

The current epoch that we are transitioning from is of war, deception and greed into an epoch of peace, truth and altruistic lovingkindness. The lessons of GOOD and EVIL are not as easy to learn as the other dualities within this realm, such as light and dark or hot and cold. This lesson of GOOD and EVIL has taken thousands of years for entities to grasp, learn and make choices based in FREE WILL.

Imagine that it only takes a 51% effort to find the Light through SERVICE to OTHERS, but, alternately, it takes a 95% effort to find the DARKNESS through SERVICE TO SELF. Those who do not make the choice, or are unable to realize the effort needed, will find themselves in the middle regions only to play the game again within this third OCTAVE. They will continue to play the game until they have knowledge of, and can make the choice between, Light and DARKNESS.

While both are paths of experience that the ONE has set before entities in this 'Path of Being', the true Light of the UNITY of ONE resides in altruistic lovingkindness. It is only through SERVICE to OTHERS that an entity can find their way back to the Original Soul, the ONE.

The fourth OCTAVE is a separation of realms into either a positively or a negatively charged experience.

The path of SERVICE to OTHERS is the path of Light, or Love and Understanding for Other-Self. The path of SERVICE to SELF is the path of DARKNESS, or Love and Understanding of Self. The positively charged path of Light is expansive. The negatively charged path of DARKNESS collapses, eventually, into SELF with no path back to the Original Soul.

The fifth OCTAVE is a continued separation into the positive expansion of Light and the negative collapsing of DARKNESS. Entities within both paths are pondering the Logic and Wisdom of their 'Path of Being' through the previous OCTAVES. Still individual entities, they are trying to resolve their potentiality, either that of Light or DARKNESS.

The sixth OCTAVE is the adjoining of individual entities into groups of positively charged BEINGS. As the negatively charged entity has no course but to collapse into nothingness within the fifth OCTAVE of DARKNESS, there is not a sixth OCTAVE of DARKNESS, only that of Light.

It is within this sixth OCTAVE that entities take their first step into true UNITY in preparation of the rejoining with the Original Soul, or the ONE. It is within this OCTAVE that the entities continue their work to resolve the 'Path of Being' that they have taken throughout the earlier OCTAVES. It is within this OCTAVE that the adjoined learn the lessons of Light and LOVE for All.

This adjoining of entities works through the choices in Free Will that each have taken with a greater understanding of how those choices have affected the Unity of ONE. It is within this sixth OCTAVE that entities make reparations for choices that have negatively affected the Unity.

The seventh OCTAVE is the great adjoining of Light. It is within this realm that entities are brought together in final preparation for the their final journey back to UNITY with the ONE. While these entities have successfully transcended all other OCTAVES, their final preparation is in losing the SEPARATION, or individualism, as they will be once again absorbed into the pure Light and LOVE of the ONE.

The eighth OCTAVE is the end of the 'Path of Being', which is as the beginning. It is in this final OCTAVE that all individual entities who have had SEPARATION join hands again within the Original Soul, the ONE.

Chapter 4
Within

The quote from the "Book of John" earlier, is a pretty bold statement. It starts with 'Behold' and ends with a pretty racy statement for the time.

"For behold, the Kingdom of God is within you."

Heaven is within you, me and everyone on the face of the Earth. At the core of our Temple is a connection to the Divine. The unseen energies, auras and Light all stem from the ONE. We connect with this source of all things from within.

Earlier I talked of the energy centers, or Chakras as they are commonly known. It is the design of our Temple. And, as such, many ancient religious texts hold these truths.

Unfortunately, these truths have been denied by many of these religions through a contradictory dogma.

In Judaism, the Menorah was one of the first teaching tools for these energy centers. The original Menorah design given to Moses and Aaron was a candelabra with seven flames in a semi-circular pattern. This was intended to teach about the energy centers.

One of the most curious tools used to teach about the energy centers is found in the Christian "Book of Revelation". Christianity, for the most part, denies these energy centers. Yet, the 'Revelation' that John had was that Heaven was 'within' him. Not only that, but he also wrote about the journey within and HOW to do it.

John used the symbols of Angels, churches, stars and other devices to teach the lessons about the energy centers. Along the way, as the energy centers are opened, there are also rewards that Spirit will give you as you continue your journey.

For instance, after the third church of Pergamum, the person will receive 'some of the hidden manna' and 'a white stone with a new name written on it'. The 'hidden manna' is that unseen energy. The 'name' that you are given is your true Spiritual name.

This church of Pergamum relates to the third Chakra, or the Solar Plexus. This Chakra is the fire of the ego, our individuality that need to be balanced. When we do, we find our true name. This energy center also opens up the top energy centers. By removing blockages in this Chakra, you get 'some' of the connection to the heavens.

And, after all of the Angels of the churches are satisfied, John relates that he was now in 'Spirit'. John took the journey within and found the 'Kingdom of God'. Along the way, he unlocked mysteries that are very much like those found within the other explanations of these energy centers from very removed and divergent ancient texts.

The system of the Chakras have been known for thousands of years. The ancient Hindu Sanskrit texts talk about these in detail. And, in that system, when you have opened all of your Chakras, you connect with the Source.

(I talk about a method of opening these energy centers in the second chapter of this book.)

As I took my journey within, Spirit opened up many great Gifts to me. Not only was I blessed with a tremendous healing vibration, I began to connect with Spirit in many amazing ways.

At first, there was a great deal of intuition. I started to clear Karma. Then, from what I understand, I began to tap into the Akashic Records.

Then I began to write my books. I tapped into the Source for much of the knowledge I share. While very esoteric at times, I have had to learn to put it into a vernacular that people could understand.

Yet, Spirit only gave me as much as I could handle. Little by little more was given to me. Currently, my Veil is just about gone.

After my 2nd Reiki Attunement, the 'Kingdom' within became clearer.

I received my 'name'. I began to talk with my guides. I tapped further into the Akashic Records. My 'healing' abilities are much stronger. I can connect with my Higher Self and fly through the Heavens.

One of the Gifts of Spirit that I received was an ability to understand a person's Octave and their 'Angel Record', as I call it.

The 'Angel Record' is the journey that a soul-being takes through this Realm of the Earth. Depending on the Octave, or Vibrational level, every soul-being's Angel Record has 7 Karmic incarnations. These 7 Karmic incarnations decide to which Octave you will ascend after your time in the Realm of the Earth.

If you are an Angel of the 7th Octave, you also have 18 'Purpose' incarnations.

Along with these incarnations, each soul-being has a number of other incarnations within this Realm that are about learning, loving and experiencing life here. These additional incarnations are based on your Vibrational level. The Angels that are here of the 3rd Octave have fewer incarnations than those of the highest Vibrational 7th Octave Angels.

These are my gifts.

I have been given them so that I can share these secrets of the ONE with you.

I stated at the beginning of this book that I am writing it to help everyone on their journey to Spirit and the ULE. It is the 'Knowledge' and 'Compassion' I hold that helps me within Reiki, and my life.

This 'Knowledge' and 'Compassion' has made my journey powerful and amazing.

I share it with you so that you can have a powerful and amazing journey in Reiki, Spirit or throughout your life.

To help you on your journey 'within', I have included a powerful meditation in Appendix B.

I use this meditation in my 'Ascension Workshops' so that people can connect to their 7 Karmic incarnations to clear their Karma, learn their lessons and cut their cords.

You can use this meditation yourself to connect to your higher self and begin your journey of self discovery.

When you use this meditation, be sure to make your intention clear when you first begin to meditate. A statement like, "I would like to connect with my other Karmic incarnations so that I might clear my Karma and learn those lessons" would be a good, specific intention.

Open yourself up to Spirit and listen. You will be guided to the work that you need to do. Don't try to force it, just let it happen.

The ONE has nothing but Light and Love waiting for you!

Chapter 5
Reiki

The origins of Reiki, and what Reiki is, are highly debated at times. There are many who want to take credit for 'discovering' Reiki. Yet, Reiki cannot be owned, controlled or even sold. Reiki is at the core of all living. Reiki, or the Universal Life Energy (ULE), has been part of existence since the first emanations.

The 'Reiki' system that I know, and have been initiated into, is Usui Reiki. I am of the Takata Sensei lineage. It is this form of Reiki that this history is told.

Usui Reiki, the modernized form of Reiki popularized throughout the world, was developed in the 1920's by a Japanese born Buddhist monk, Dr. Mikao Usui, Usui Sensei. While teaching in a college, Dr. Usui was asked by a student how Jesus facilitated the healing miracles that he performed. The question had planted a seed and set Dr. Usui out on the path to answer that question. Dr. Usui was determined to learn the secret healing so that he may help others. His journey took him to many countries.

At the time, there were a number of Reiki systems available in Japan. Dr. Usui was familiar with them. Each had it's own system of healing and teaching.

Dr. Usui began a journey of discovering Reiki for himself.

During his journey Dr Usui traveled to the holy mountains of Kori Yama where he fasted and meditated for 21 days in order to attain a high altered state of consciousness. He believed this would empower him with the healing energy. On the morning of the 21st day, Dr. Usui was beginning to become frustrated with his situation. As he was about to give up and leave, a great spiritual energy came down into the top of his head and he became enlightened. The energy bought with it Reiki Ryoho, which is the ability to heal.

For Usui Sensei, Reiki was a spiritual practice – an opportunity for each person to awaken their true nature.

From the inscription on Usui Sensei's memorial stone, "The number of pupils who learned from Usui Sensei amounts to more than 2000 persons. Some leading pupils living in Tokyo among them gather at the training center and take over his work, while other pupils in the country also do everything to popularize the REIKI cure."

One of Usui Sensei's pupils was Dr Chujiro Hayashi who continued in the steps of Usui Sensei by opening a Reiki clinic which remained opened until 1940. He became a student of Usui Sensei in May 1925 and is one of the twenty one teacher students of Usui Sensei. He was a retired Naval Officer and surgeon and he studied with Usui Sensei for 10 months before Usui Sensei transitioned in March 1926.

Dr Hayashi developed a new style of Reiki, which has the same energy and lineage as Usui Reiki, and many of the original techniques. Hayashi Sensei is also responsible for the formal aspects of Reiki which are taught today – namely the hand positions, the science-based practices held within Reiki and an 'attunement'.

The fame and popularity of Hayashi Sensei's clinic spread throughout Japan, and it was quite successful at bringing the healing energies of Reiki to many people. In Dr. Hayashi's clinic the emphasis was on healing rather than personal development.

Mrs. Hawayo Takata was a Hawaiian woman of Japanese descent born in 1900. After the death of her husband and sister, she became sick and decided to travel to Japan in search of a doctor who could perform an operation which was deemed necessary in order for her good health to return.

While in Japan, she felt strongly that the operation would be unnecessary, and she inquired if there was any alternative way for her to be healed. The doctor referred her to Dr Hayashi's clinic.

Mrs. Takata began receiving regular weekly treatments. Over a period of several weeks, her health improved drastically.

She was amazed and asked Dr Hayashi to teach her how to transmit Reiki energies to others. He agreed to teach her Reiki I and II and she studied with him from 1936 to 1938. She is one of the thirteen teacher students of Hayashi Sensei.

She was the first to bring Hayashi Sensei's teaching to the west when she returned to Hawaii where she began to practice Reiki.

Two years later, she convinced Hayashi Sensei to come visit her in Hawaii so he could see her Reiki clinic. After seeing the clinic, Hayashi Sensei decided to initiate Mrs Takata into the third degree of Reiki.

Takata Sensei continued giving treatments and began teaching level 1 and level 2 Reiki students.

In the 1970's, she began training other Reiki masters. For over 40 years she used storytelling to teach people about the system she called Reiki and its history.

By the time of her transition on December 11th 1980, Takata Sensei had trained 22 Reiki masters. It is mainly from these teachers that Usui Reiki has spread throughout the west.

Takata Sensei's 22 Reiki Masters:

George Araki
Dorothy Baba
Ursula Baylow
Rick Bockner
Patricia Bowling
Barbara Brown
Fran Brown
Phyllis Furumoto
Beth Gray
John Gray

Iris Ishikuro
Harry Kuboi
Ethel Lombardi
Barbara McCullough
Mary McFadyen
Paul Mitchell
Bethel Phaigh
Shinobu Saito
Virginia Samdahl
Wanja Twan
Barbara Weber Ray
Kay Yamashita

From these 22 Reiki Masters most of the world knows about Reiki.

Currently, there are thousands of Reiki Masters worldwide. Many hold the traditions that came to the West by Takata Sensei's teachings.

I am 9[h] in line to Usui Sensei through the lineage of Takata Sensei.

Soon, I too will be able to teach Reiki through the traditions of my Reiki Masters. That is not something I take lightly or can do through this book

Yet, that is not the full story of Reiki. That is just the story of Usui Reiki's discovery and modernization by Usui Sensei.

As stated earlier, Reiki is a system of being a channel for the ULE. These systems have been around since the dawn of man, as this Light is woven within us.

In the Hindu tradition, the Light is called 'Prana'. In Hindu philosophy including yoga, Indian medicine and martial arts, Prana (the Sanskrit word for "life force" or "vital principle") comprises all cosmic energies that permeate the Universe on all levels.

In the Chinese tradition, the Light is called 'Qi' or 'Chi'. Chi is a Chinese word meaning aliveness, life force energy. or life breath.

The Definition of Chi: "Theories of traditional Chinese medicine assert that the body has natural patterns of qi associated with it that circulate in channels called meridians in English.

In Reiki, one is taught that it is the seven main energy centers, or Chakras, that primarily facilitate the flow of energy through the body. While there are minor Chakras within the body, the hand positions for most Reiki traditions correspond to these main energy centers.

When a Reiki practitioner 'Heals' a client, they are really just becoming a channel for the Light, removing blockages within the client, and facilitating the proper flow of Light so the client can heal themselves.

The Usui Reiki that originated from Takata Sensei has 3 levels of initiation, or 'attunements', as shown to her from Hayashi Sensei.

The 1st Degree opens you up to the Reiki.

The 2nd Degree gives you the Power, Emotional and Distant/Physical symbols to use during healings.

The 3rd Degree, or Reiki Master, allows you to teach and gives you the Master symbol to use.

Yet, that is only the system of Reiki that is handed down from Master to student in my lineage.

Reiki is uniquely individual. As each of us is attuned to the Light differently. When you are opened up to the Light, the three natures of the ONE show differently in everyone.

Yet, you will only be given as much as you can handle.

In my experience of opening up to the Light, my gifts of the ONE have been amazing.

After the 1st initiation, I was slowly opened up to a greater healing and a type of omniscient gift. It seems I have been able to tap into the Akashic Records.

After my 2nd initiation, all three natures opened up to me. I learned I could peer into the past and future. It was easier for me to go into meditation and do distant healing. I also found I could 'fly' by a form of astral projection. And, the flow of Light increased within me, I was given a greater understanding of Reiki healing, both local and distant.

Chapter 6
Physical

In Reiki we learn how to clear ourselves and create the space for people so that the Light can flow into them for healing. Reiki practitioners do not diagnose, treat or do anything to their clients other than channel the Light. The Light does the healing. The client's own Temple assists the healing.

Sometimes, Reiki practitioner is guided by intuition to place a Power, Emotional or Distant/Physical sign into a blockage to help release it. But, it is the client who does the releasing. It is the client who must learn the lesson involved.

Sometimes, there are Karmic influences that take more work to release than simply a few Reiki treatments. These may be past life lessons that were never learned or which are currently playing out. A Reiki practitioner can assist with these blockages, but ultimately it is the client that needs to work them out.

When I started healing regularly, I worked in a Spiritual clinic that offered free Reiki healing every Wednesday evening. There were usually 5 Reiki practitioners working and we typically saw upwards of 8 to 10 people each.

This was great practice for me. Each one of these free healings only lasted about 10 or 15 minutes, but I was able to do some great work in that time. There were many instances when I would see the people again and they commented on the energies they received.

Many of these people suffered from the stress and emotional dysfunction of modern life. I typically knew if I needed to work on the persons emotional or physical centers, or if they just needed a good shot of Light. For the most part, I would quickly open up the Chakras and make sure the Light was flowing in them.

One afternoon when I was setting up, I walked into the lobby where people were waiting. I scanned the crowd and saw a woman who I thought looked familiar. I half waved and turned around as I realized I had never met her.

During these free Reiki healings, the clients put their name on a list. I never know who I am going to get, as it is pretty random. When you are ready to heal a client, you take the next person on the list.

Well, I finished setting up and went back into the lobby to get my first client. I looked on the list and called out the next name, "Becky".

To my surprise, it was the woman I saw earlier. I greeted her and led her back to my treatment room.

This was Becky's first time at the clinic and first time receiving Reiki, so I explained the process to her. I then asked her to lay down on the table and relax.

I then began my Reiki session, calling in my Guides.

Almost as soon as I started to work on Becky, she began to raise her hands in the air. I sensed that the energies she was sensing was too much for her. So, I asked about it.

She told me that about four weeks prior, these energies pretty much overtook her. They came on all of a sudden and she really didn't know what to make of them.

I continued the treatment and realized there was probably something Karmic going on with her. I settled the energies down for her by opening her Chakras and by giving her the emotional symbol, but I knew I wasn't finished.

After the treatment, Becky had a large emotional release. So, I talked with her for a bit and asked her about her Spiritual journey. I inquired more about her energies.

I knew she needed a full Reiki session to open up the major emotional block I sensed.

I realized what Karmic block Becky had, but I knew that she was not ready to hear it. She descended from the 7th Octave into this Realm. Her blockage was from what I call the events of year '0'. This was the time of Jesus. I sensed that Becky was there in a past life and her blockage/awakening had something to do with that.

I was concerned for her. She was experiencing energies that most people don't feel until after their 2nd Reiki initiation. I gave her my number and asked her to text me if there was any changes.

The next day Becky contacted me.

She stated that she was fine when she left, but went to a friends house and got out of balance again. It seems her friends know about the energies, but play in Spirit blindly. Her association with these individuals messes with her energies somehow.

I knew Becky needed a full Reiki treatment, so I scheduled it with her the next day.

When Becky arrived, I had already prepared for her. My treatment table was set up and I took out my tools to read her Angel Record.

I sat her down and quickly explained the Path of Being. I did her Angel Record and showed her the 18 incarnations of purpose she has because of her descending from the 7th Octave and how her Karma is tied into it. I explained that she lived in the time of Jesus, was one of his followers and saw him die on the cross.

Becky's emotional blockage was that of witnessing the punishment of Jesus and feeling like she failed him.

With just this knowledge, I felt Becky was on the road to removing that blockage. I knew that when I put her on the table, it would be easier for her to release it.

So, I had her lay down and relax.

I began at her head and placed my hands over her eyes. I felt her pulling energy from my hands. I placed the Emotional symbol in her Crown then put the Power Symbol in.

I then moved my hands to her ears, under her head, then to her Heart Chakra. It was at her Heart Chakra that I felt the most pull.

I then put the Distant/Physical, Emotional and Power symbols directly into her Chakra. I let the energy flow into this blockage.

Soon, both Becky and I felt the blockage begin to move up to her Crown and out. I told her to just relax and let it go. She unlocked the blockage and I helped push it out.

I then sealed up her wound and moved on.

I then went to her Lower Chakras, one by one. By the time I got to her feet, I felt the balance return to her. I finished her with another Power symbol to seal her and began to cleanse her Aura.

After the treatment, Becky told me how good she felt.

She went on her way that night thinking it was over, but I knew that the release would be soon. I was right.

I got a text from Becky that she opened up when she got home and started crying. I told her to just let it out. She did and thanked me.

The next morning, I wanted to see how Becky was doing and make sure her wound was healed.

I prepared to meditate so that I could visit Becky remotely and do a Distant Healing for her.

Chapter 7
Distance

In Reiki we also learn how to do Distant healing. The Distance/Physical Reiki symbol that you are given in your second initiation means 'No past, present, future'. It is also a very powerful symbol for physical healing.

There have been many times when I have done Distant healing with Reiki. And, each time I do it, I am amazed at the process and outcome. Most of the time, the recipient feels the treatment and is positively affected by a distant healing.

With Becky, I knew that I needed to check the treatment I gave her the day before. While most practitioners only do one treatment for a person, my lineage believes that a person should have four initial treatments.

So, in the morning, I visited Becky remotely.

The first step I take in distant healing is the same I take in deep meditation or distant viewing – I ground myself very well.

I always use the meditation in 'Appendix B'. Again, I will use the grounding and ascension within this meditation, but the intention I use is 'Healing'. The clearer and concise the intention is the better.

After I ground myself and ascend into Spirit, I begin the Distant Reiki healing.

The first step is to call my Guides in and then contact Becky's for permission to do the Distant healing treatment. Everyone agreed and I began. If they didn't agree to the healing, I would respectively cut the session right there.

During a Distant healing, the first thing I notice when I enter the client's subtle energy body is their energy signature. I see whether their Chakras are open, where potential blockages are and the unique energy signature of the Angel within.

With Becky, her energy was up, but I noticed a dark mass still in her heart. I proceeded to help Becky heal and seal this blockage.

While in the Distant healing, I still use the hand positions and the process that I use in my regular Reiki healings.

I started at Becky's head and placed my two hands over the representation of her eyes in my 'mind's eye'. Even though I am doing the healing remotely, I still feel the pull of energy through my Crown to my hands. Becky was pulling a good bit of Light today.

As I held my hands above her eyes, I sent her the Distant/Physical symbol to begin. I immediately felt an evening of the pull from Becky As I knew this blockage was emotional, I also sent her that symbol. I then pushed the Power symbol through my hands.

As I felt the energies balance, I moved my hands.

Well, not literally, as I was still in my mind's eye doing the Distant healing.

I moved my hands to the side of Becky's head, just over where her ears would be. I stayed in that position for a couple of minutes and let the Light flow.

I then moved to the back of Becky's head, to her throat and then onto her heart. For each area I try to spend a couple of minutes sending the area Light.

When I moved to Becky's heart, I felt a strong pull through my right hand, which would be her left side. At this point I knew I was right over the Karmic blockage.

Keeping my hands over Becky's heart, I placed the three Reiki symbols into this blockage. I held my hands over this spot, moving my left hand from it's normal position. I held my hands until I felt the blockage seal.

Once I sensed this Karmic wound heal, I placed another Power symbol over it as a sort of bandage. At this point the wound had turned light from dark.

I felt confident at this point that Becky's Karmic wound from the year '0' was healed.

I then moved my hands down Becky to her Solar Plexus, Sacral, and Root Chakras. On each of these I stayed for a couple of minutes.

I then moved my hands to her knees and then down to her feet. I finished Becky's Distant healing by placing a Power symbol into the soles of her feet. I then waited until I felt the Light was flowing smoothly within Becky.

At the end of the Distant treatment I thank all of the Guides, both Becky's and mine, then close the connection.

As this Distant healing took place in the morning, I waited a few hours to contact Becky to see if there was any change. I wanted to give the Light enough time to do their work.

After a few hours, I sent Becky a text and asked her how she was doing. Her answer really didn't surprise me.

Becky told me she woke up a bit groggy. She then shared that she had a bit of an emotional release a couple of hours ago. I inquired how she felt now. Becky stated she felt great after her rough morning.

I've never heard from Becky again.

And, that's the way it usually goes when you are a Light worker. People usually enter your life when they need the special services or relationship that only you can give. And, by relationship, I mean a Karmic tie that the two of you may not even be aware of.

My interaction with Becky was solely for the removal of that Karmic wound. It is not for me to understand the why or how, but to only provide my unique gifts of Spirit.

Since I have started really working the Light within Reiki, the Three Natures of Spirit have manifested in amazing ways. From the omnipotent, omnipresent and omniscient I have begun healing within the Light in far more ways than just traditional Reiki.

And, my journey is just beginning.

Chapter 8
Journey

While my spiritual journey has introduced me to Reiki, Reiki has introduced me to Spirit in so many amazing ways. The more that I feel the Light flow through my body, the greater are the Gifts of Spirit bestowed upon me.

And, these Gifts can be yours as well.

These Gifts of Spirit, the omnipotent, omnipresent and the omniscient are precious abilities that we all have available to us. Every single person upon the Earth can access these Gifts of Spirit.

It is truly our design.

As our bodies allow the flow of Light, this Light brings with it a remarkable healing power. As these Gifts of Spirit are inherent abilities within us, the removal of the blockages in Reiki allow the Light to flow, they also allow the Gifts of Spirit a chance to blossom.

Are these gifts a by-product of Reiki?

Well, yes and no.

These Gifts of Spirit are a product of the Light and Love of the ONE. As we move closer to the Light, these gifts are bestowed that we might heal on a greater level.

And, that is exactly what I do.

I use Reiki to unblock MYSELF so that I might be a channel to the Light. The more the Light flows through me, the greater my Gifts of Spirit manifest. And, as I continue to remove the blockages, these Gifts grow.

So, in that sense, yes, Gifts of Spirit are a by-product of being initiated into Reiki. When you are initiated into Reiki, major blockages are seemingly removed quickly as each initiation opens the pathways of Light within you.

Reiki is a fast track to remove blockages and allow the Light to move freely throughout yourself.

The normal track, which is not to say it is the 'slow' track, is the more natural or organic way to remove blockages. This is done by doing exercises, meditation and self-discovery.

Yet, it seems, many of life's greatest lessons are Karmic in nature and appear in our lives when they are meant to be. And, until these Karmic lessons surface, we can only wait and hope our self-discovery helps resolve these situations.

I learned long ago that 'to know oneself, one has to find oneself'. My journey in Reiki is really a journey to find myself.

Since a very early age, I have known that there was something more to life. I felt a bit out of place in the world that my parents accepted.

For as long as I can remember, I searched for clues. I looked within books, manuscripts and ancient reliefs. I looked within ancient religions and traditions.

Then, one day, I believed I found the answer – the Light.

In a quest to find the Light, I discovered Reiki.

Reiki is seemingly the only system that recognizes and works with the Light – in all of existence.

That is not to say that other traditions and systems aren't using the Light to heal. It's just that Reiki is the only system that I have found which seeks to understand the unexplainable through a science-based process easy enough for anyone to understand and learn.

My journey to find the Light in Reiki started in 2001. I don't know if I was really ready for Reiki, but it seems Reiki was ready for me. I have always been somewhat of a healer, so I thought that Reiki would strengthen the energies everyone said I had.

Yet, I didn't use Reiki consistently for the first decade after getting my first Reiki initiation. While I gave family and friends massages and energy work, it was just a normal part of who I was.

What I didn't realize is that the Light was slowly building and flowing smoother through me even though I did not practice Reiki regularly.

I started to really notice the Gifts of Spirit when a different Reiki Master gave me the 1st Degree initiation again and the 2nd Degree initiation for the first time.

The 2nd Degree initiation must have opened some major blockages in me. That was my first experience with the Distance/Physical symbol. That symbol means 'No past, no present and no future'.

Ever since this 2nd Degree Reiki initiation, the Akashic Records have been opened to me. Through being able to access this knowledge, I have been able to see my many incarnations within this Realm.

Yes, I can see many of my past, present and future lives.

Not only my incarnations within this Realm, but anyone's. I can see the date of their incarnation as well as the place. And, I can see which Octave they have descended from and will ascend too.

I call these our "Angel Record".

This has also strengthened much of my other works. While I have done dozens of "Angel Records", they verify some of the other conceptual understandings of Spirit, this Realm and the ONE.

But, that is only one of the Gifts of Spirit I have unlocked since starting to practice Reiki.

I now have a new Reiki Master, or Sensei, that will give me my Reiki Master initiation.

While there are some differences in the Reiki lineage, I chose to take all three initiations in this new lineage. To honor and understand fully, my choice for a new Sensei was on doing all three initiations again.

So, I took the initiations for the first two Reiki Degrees again from my new Sensei. The first one was on a beach in Florida. The second was on a river bank.

Even though I had already been initiated into the first two degrees of Reiki, the 1st and 2nd Degree under this new Reiki lineage was very powerful.

My current Reiki lineage does distant healing a little differently than my first. My first lineage uses a 'proxy', like a teddy bear, while the second imagines the client in between the hands. I find this new way of distant healing very powerful for me, as in Becky's case of the last couple chapters.

I personally find my new Reiki lineage and their techniques to be very powerful – to me.

And, that is the journey – self-discovery.

Your journey to find Reiki will be far different than mine. And, that is perfect, for your journey will unblock the Light in ways that only you can discover.

I fully believe in the power of Reiki to heal.

And, that healing has taken form in my life in so many ways. It all began with hands on Reiki healing. Then it moved to Distant Healing.

And, in between the Gifts of Spirit grew in me and inspired me to write a number of books. I then begin reading people's "Angel Record" to heal Karmic ties.

Right now I am sitting on a mountain in Salida, Colorado writing this book and awaiting my initiation as Reiki Master. I will still be in training for the next year to teach others Reiki, but it is well worth it.

I just hope this short book has given you an insight into Reiki so that you might be strong in your journey.

The "Knowledge" and "Compassion" that I share in this book is universal. I hope that it helps you in your life whether you take a Reiki journey, or not.

My journey is really just beginning.

Appendix A
Tree of Life

The "Tree of Life" is a poem by a 16th Century Judaic Rabbi Isaac Luria. He is considered the father of contemporary Kabbalah. His teachings are referred to as Lurianic Kabbalah.

While his direct literary contribution to the Kabbalistic school of Safed was extremely minute (he wrote only a few poems), his spiritual fame led to their veneration and the acceptance of his authority. The works of his disciples compiled his oral teachings into writing.

The "Tree of Life" is one of Isaac Luria's amazing poems that seeks to explain the Light, Creation and our place within the ONE.

Tree of Life
by Isaac Luria

behold
that before the emanations were emanated
and the creatures created,
the upper simple light had filled
the whole existence.
And there was no vacancy,

such as an empty atmosphere,
a hollow, or a pit.
But all was filled
with simple, boundless light.
And there was no such part
as head, or tail.
But everything was simple,
smooth light,
balanced evenly and equally,
And it was called
the Endless Light.
And when upon His simple will,
came the desire to create the world
and emanate the emanations,
to bring to light the perfection
of His deeds,
His names, His appellations,
which was the cause
of the creation of the worlds,
He then restricted Himself, in the middle,
precisely in the center,
He restricted the light.
And the light drew far off to the sides
around that middle point.
and there remained an empty space,
a vacuum
circling he middle point.
And the restriction had been uniform
around the empty point,

so that the space
was evenly circled around it.
There, after the restriction,
having formed a vacuum and a space
precisely in the middle of the endless light,
a place was formed
where the emanated
and the created
might reside.
Then from Endless Light
a single line hung down,
lowered down into that space,
and through that line,
He emanated, formed,
created all the worlds.
Before these four worlds came to be
there was one infinite,
one name,
in wondrous, hidden
unity,
that even for the closest of the angels
there is no attainment in the endless.
as there is no mind that can perceive it
for He has
no place,
no boundary
no name

Appendix B
Meditation

This meditation is very grounding and powerful.

Find a nice quiet place, sit comfortably with feet firmly planted in front of you with your palms up on your lap

Close your eyes and relax

Breath in slowly and fill your lungs, hold it

Now slowly breath out through your mouth

Breath in

Breath out

Now, as you breath in, feel the energy come in through crown

As you breath out, send it down through your body

Feel the energy as you push it past your feet and into the Earth

Ground yourself in the Earth with the energy

With each breath you take, push it further into the Earth - to the center

Now, bring the energy of the Earth back up into your feet

Feel it go through and awaken your base Chakra with the red glow

Feel it go through and awaken your Sacral Chakra with the Orange glow

Feel it go through and awaken your Solar Plexus Chakra with the Yellow glow

Feel it go through and awaken your Heart Chakra with the Green glow of love

Feel it go through and awaken your Throat Chakra with the blue glow of communication

Feel it go through and awaken your Third Eye Chakra with the Violet glow of awareness

Feel it go through and awaken your Crown Chakra with the white glow of your connection to your higher self

You feel your Crown Chakra connecting to the Heavenly realms and to your higher self

You now follow that stream of energy up, out of your body and in to the Heavens above

You slowly float up, rising above this building and into the sky

Now approaching the clouds, you slow your ascent and rest upon a cloud

The stream of energy to your higher self still travels up but you rest here, still in the realm of the Earth.

(Now this is where I put the intention. It is your job to ask for guidance or specific requests, like: answers to questions, talking with guides or loved ones, cutting Karmic cords, or something else you may need)

(In my 'Ascension Workshop', I use this intention.)

Ask your higher self to send down your other 6 Karmic incarnations.

Slowly, six others sit with you on the cloud.

Talk, reconcile, forgive.

Cut the cords of Karma from these past lives.

Remove those things that do not serve your Higher Self, those things you need not hold.

Forgive yourself, forgive the past, and find peace to love yourself.

Sit there for a while and work these Karmic lessons out so that you may remove any blockages to the Light you may unnecessarily hold.

(let 5 minutes go by and bring back)

Now thank your Higher Self. Cut the cords of any vows or agreements that you made within these Karmic lives, for these should not be held by you in this incarnation.

Be at peace with your past.

Be at peace with yourself.

Now, begin your descent back to your physical body.

As you settle in, bring the stream of your Higher Self back down.

Pull the anchor up that you have in the Earth.

Slowly begin to move.

When you are ready, open your eyes.

You are now back full physical within this current incarnation.

Appendix C
Sevenfold Teaching

The First Understanding in Truth is:
All of Creation is ONE; is ONE entity; is the ONE.

The Second Understanding in Truth is:
The ONE is the Creator; by whose Word all of Creation exists as the ONE.

The Third Understanding in Truth is:
The ONE is holy; as Creation is holy; as you are holy.

The Fourth Understanding in Truth is:
All are ONE in unity; ONE with each other in unity.

The Fifth Understanding in Truth is:
The heart of the ONE is altruistic lovingkindness; as should yours be.

The Sixth Understanding in Truth is:
Give of yourselves in service to the ONE; to Creation; to each other.

The Seventh Understanding in Truth is:
In this moment there is only the love of the ONE.

From "Sevenfold Teaching" by Mark F. Kalita 2012

Appendix D
Protection

As you are now working in the Light, you must also be aware that there is darkness that doesn't like the Light. You should learn how to protect and shield yourself from the darkness.

This is a very powerful, simple prayer that I find works at keeping me protected from the darkness. Sometimes, I extend the prayer with things like 'cleanse me' or 'allow me to do your will'. Those additions are not needed for this prayer to work. I just do that to remind me of my purpose in the Light of ONE.

Prayer of Archangel Mika'el

As I stand in this moment of Unity with ALL,
giving thanks and praise to the ONE,
I ask that you bless me
and envelope me in your Light,
that you will be with me to keep me from evil
so that I cause no pain.

About the Author

Mark F. Kalita is the author of over 40 books on Spirituality and our Spiritual nature. Mark believes that it is his purpose in life to transfer this knowledge of the Ascensions and the Light of the Angelic Realm to our People.

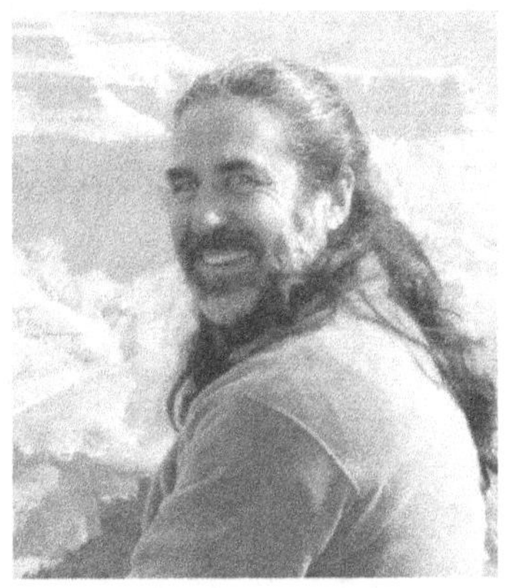

Besides his role as Author, Mark also teaches workshops such as the "Ascension Workshop". With interests in Tarot, Crystals, Healing and other Spiritual Gifts, Mark wants to share his knowledge with others.

When Mark isn't writing or teaching, he spends time outdoors planting or planning gardens. His vision is to create a vast wilderness of food to provide sustenance for our People. From fruit bearing trees to herbs and edibles, Mark's dream is to create a new epoch of lovingkindness in which all of our basic needs are met – beginning with food!

Each new story Mark creates is an inspirational bridge to a world that could be. A world without suffering. A world bathed in the Light of knowledge and compassion founded in the Unity of Existence.

Other books by
Mark F. Kalita

These and other books can all be found at:

www.KALITA.com

Or, through Amazon in paperback or Kindle